CARNIVORE DIET

Your Complete Guide to
the Carnivore Diet and Complete Meal Plans

Susan Grey

© Copyright 2019 by Susan Grey All rights reserved.

This document is geared towards providing exact and reliable information in regards to the topic and issue covered. The publication is sold with the idea that the publisher is not required to render accounting, officially permitted, or otherwise, qualified services. If advice is necessary, legal or professional, a practiced individual in the profession should be ordered.

- From a Declaration of Principles which was accepted and approved equally by a Committee of the American Bar Association and a Committee of Publishers and Associations.

In no way is it legal to reproduce, duplicate, or transmit any part of this document in either electronic means or in printed format. Recording of this publication is strictly prohibited and any storage of this document is not allowed unless with written permission from the publisher. All rights reserved.

The information provided herein is stated to be truthful and consistent, in that any liability, in terms of inattention or otherwise, by any usage or abuse of any policies, processes, or directions contained within is the solitary and utter responsibility of the recipient reader. Under no circumstances will any legal responsibility or blame be held against the publisher for any reparation, damages, or monetary loss due to the information herein, either directly or indirectly.

Respective authors own all copyrights not held by the publisher.

The information herein is offered for informational purposes solely, and is universal as so. The presentation of the information is without contract or any type of guarantee assurance.

Grow Your Pantry Are On A Mission

To get 2,000,000 people to grow their own food over the next 10 years...

How will we help 2,000,000 people reconnect to their food?

Free online resources, affordable kitchen products, affordable growing products

For free ebooks on growing your own food, recipes and how to guides just visit our website and enter your email at:

www.growyourpantry.com

Once you've signed up to our exclusive emailing list you will receive your first free e-book!

Between our online resource centre and free content delivered to you weekly via email be sure to not miss out...

TABLE OF CONTENTS

Overview 1

Introduction 3

Health Disclaimer 3

Chapter 1: What Is The Carnivore Diet? 5
    Background Of The Carnivore Diet 8
    Considerations When Starting The Carnivore Diet 14
    Effects On Your Body 16

Chapter 2: Starter Guide 19
    What Can You Eat? 20

Chapter 3: Meal Plans & Recipes 25

Links 45

OVERVIEW

The Carnivore diet is one that is not new to mankind. There are cultures that have been eating a meat only diet for years yet we never knew about it. It is only in recent years that more and more people are seriously looking into taking up this diet, not only for short term health reasons but as a lifestyle. Although there is currently no formal research on the benefits of taking on a meat only diet, those who have turned it into a lifestyle have taken laboratory tests whose results show that their body responds better to not having any carbohydrates or plants in their diet. This goes against the conventional eating habits that we have grown up with. Since we can remember, we have been taught that one must eat a balanced diet which includes carbohydrates, proteins, vitamins and a side of fruit. Parents do their best to ensure their children eat their potato, broccoli and spinach because it is good for them. Carrots are good for your eyes, fibre is good for digestion, meat, especially red meat is bad for you.

With these eating habits drilled into us from childhood, it requires a paradigm shift of sorts to take on the carnivore diet. Either that or the desire to get some reprieve from a chronic illness. Most of the initial converts were suffering from some form of autoimmune disease and were eliminating certain foods from their diet so as to understand what triggered their illness. As they dug deeper and eliminated most foods from their diet, they discovered the carnivore diet. When they applied it, their lives turned around as almost all the symptoms of their illness subsided. It seemed that plant-based foods irritated their bodies and triggered a variety of ailments.

Anyone recovered from a debilitating disease by changing what they eat would shout about it from the rooftops. They truly appreciate what good health is and they have a different perspective on how what you eat affects your body. However, one may argue that these are isolated and individual experiences and should not be used to advocate for the carnivore diet. More so as it has not been thoroughly researched and proven to be beneficial to those who are seemingly healthy.

Why would one want to switch from their omnivorous diet to a purely carnivorous diet yet they have been doing quite well healthwise? This is where individual preference comes into play. If you are content with your level of health and fitness yet are willing to experiment, you are welcome to try out the carnivore diet and see how it works for you. For those seeking higher levels of health, or those seeking to understand how different foods affect one's body, trying out the carnivore diet is part of taking your health to the next level.

The carnivore diet can be broken down into various levels. For those starting out, it is recommended to start with meat, fish, animal products which include eggs, dairy, and to keep your tea, coffee and any supplements. Stick to this level for about 30 days to see how your body responds, and to help you determine if you want to take it to the next level, if you have had enough, or if you are content to stop and go back to your regular diet. The second level eliminates all processed meats, animal products, tea and coffee. At the top, there is a strict carnivore diet where you eat nothing but meat with salt and drink just water. Again, after 30 days, one has the option to slowly begin to reintroduce the eliminated foods to see how the body responds, or just stick to that level of the carnivore diet. As a precaution, one needs to follow the recommended guidelines otherwise they will be doing the diet wrong which may have an adverse effect on their health, or not produce the expected results. Ultimately, it is an individual decision as to what level of the carnivore diet one will take up, for how long, and what outcomes one expect to see at the end of the diet.

This ebook provides a basic introduction to the carnivore diet. It looks at the background of the diet, what the benefits are, the effects on your body, and how and what to eat.

Full Legal Disclaimer

HEALTH DISCLAIMER
Last updated March 19 2019

Introduction

The information contained in the Carnivore Diet Ebook is for the provision of general instruction and informational purposes only. The information herein has been put together in good faith, however, the authors make no representation or warranty of any kind, express or implied, regarding the validity, adequacy, reliability, availability or applicability of any information provided inside the Carnivore Diet Ebook.

Under no circumstance shall we carry any liability on behalf of the reader with regard to any loss or damage of any kind that may occur as a result of the use of the ebook or application of any information given inside the ebook. The use of the ebook and your dependence on any information provided inside the ebook is done solely at your own risk.

Health Disclaimer

The Carnivore Diet Ebook does not contain health advice. The information in relation to health is provided as general information and should be used for educational purposes only and not as professional health advice.

Consequently, you are encouraged to consult with the relevant medical and/or healthcare experts before taking any actions based on the information provided in this Ebook. The Ebook does not provide any kind of health advice. Using or depending on any of the information provided inside this Ebook is done wholly at your own risk.

CARNIVORE DIET

CHAPTER 1:
What Is The Carnivore Diet?

Main Ingredients

The Carnivore diet consists of eating primarily meat or animal products. This diet is a great option for people who love meat and feel like they can eat it three times a day. Essentially, taking on the Carnivore diet means that your meal plan is filled with beef, pork, lamb, organ meats, poultry, fish, bone marrow, eggs, bone broth, and butter. There should be no vegetables, fruit or carbohydrates on your plate whatsoever. It literally means no legumes, nuts, seeds, grains, bread, pasta … you get the idea. You really get to eat meat for every meal of the day, and as much as you like.

The aim of this diet is to eliminate any plant-based products from your meals and focus on getting all your nutrients from animal products. Different parts of the animal contain different nutritional value, therefore eating different parts of a cow will provide you with a balanced diet. This means eating parts of the head, muscles, bones, tail, and organs, a concept known as eating from nose to tail.

It sounds out of this world and seems to defy conventional wisdom considering that we have been brought up knowing that a balanced diet consists of set portions of carbohydrate, protein and vitamin. If you could not remember which was which, each food group was assigned a colour to help you remember what your plate should look like. White for the carbohydrates, reddish-brown for the protein, and green for the vitamins. Carbohydrates took the largest space on the plate followed by vitamins and lastly protein. This was because we were told that protein is difficult for the body to digest, so small quantities are sufficient to meet nutritional needs. We have gone so far as to measure the number of calories and nutrients each food group contains and how much the body requires on a daily basis to run efficiently, and we follow it because we want to be healthy.

The carnivore diet pretty much throws this whole theory of a balanced diet from the different food groups out of the window. It is somewhat difficult to picture one sitting down for meal after meal, after meal of just meat! Meat for breakfast, meat for lunch, meat for dinner. This is what those who follow the diet strictly do. The eat meat and drink water. It would seem okay to do it for one meal to satisfy a craving for meat, but not on a daily basis for days on end. To be fair, eating just meat and drinking only water is not a requirement although it is highly recommended. To make it easier to adjust to the new eating habits, there are those who add their own variations to the diet to meet their personal preferences. Those who are not too strict continue to enjoy their tea and coffee, and some dairy products. However, the general guidelines are to avoid any food other than meat and other animal products. Again, this depends on one's expected outcomes after taking on the diet.

According to Diana Rodgers, RD, of the Sustainable Dish, most of the people who go on the carnivore diet do so after trying the paleo or ketogenic diet. The Paleo diet, which is also commonly known as the caveman diet requires one to stop eating added sugars, grains, dairy and legumes and eat more fresh fruits, vegetables, meats that are grass-fed and wild seafood. The ketogenic diet requirements are somewhat different as one is required to eat moderate proteins, very little carbohydrate, and a lot of fat. The carnivore diet is a step up of the two diets; simpler to follow with more refined results.

Plants Don't Want To Be Eaten

Though the carnivore diet may seem extreme in its elimination of plants and plant products, there is some research that shows that plants don't want to be eaten. While this may seem like a bias where a meat-eating diet is being promoted, the facts show that plants find ways to survive by discouraging predators from eating them. They grow thorns, secrete enzymes that make them difficult to digest or that make the predator sick, they grow in a way to hide the sweetest part or grow in hard to find places.

It may seem surreal but plants go to the extent of housing the enemies of predators to keep the predators away. An example would be the Acacia tree which attracts ants to live in an on it by producing sap that the ants like. This, in turn, makes it repulsive to herbivores. Who wants to eat or go near a plant with ants on it? The Passion flower grows its leaves with a pattern that resembles butterfly eggs. This defence mechanism keeps butterflies from laying eggs on the leaf as it seems like it is already occupied.

The seeds also have their defence mechanism as they are the main way the plant reproduces. They produce anti-nutrients that make it difficult for the human body to absorb nutrients, affect the digestive process, cause allergic reactions and food sensitivities.

On the other hand, some plants have found a way to use predators (read humans) to help them spread their seeds. Fruits for example, when unripe are not attractive at all but once ripe, smell and taste delicious and are easy to see and reach. We eat the fruits, which have laxative properties, the seeds pass through our digestive systems and are released somewhere other than where the fruit was initially picked. The fruit has won. Obviously, this worked better in the less modern ages where there was no toilet to flush, but the concept remains the same.

Human beings are very resilient and have found ways to deal with these enzymes that make plants in their various stages of growth unpalatable. We have discovered that boiling them reduces the effects of the enzymes, so does fermenting them. However, this does not mean that plants are good for us.

The Science Behind It

The all meat diet is essentially an elimination diet. Some of those who follow it started off wanting to find the remedy for an ailment or illness that was causing them a lot of distress. Research about how food affects our bodies, moods and the like, led them to identify and eliminate the offending foods from their diet. Depending on the extent of their ailment, some got to the point the only thing on their plate was meat. Others heard about the diet, and because they are interested in keeping their body healthy, decided to try it out for a couple of weeks and came away with improvements to their body that they were not expecting.

According to Paul Saladino MD, there for four key aspects to keep in mind when taking up the Carnivore diet. He breaks down the science behind how eating different parts of the animal gives you the nutrients you require to keep healthy. These are some of the nutrients that we get from eating plants but are readily available in one animal, depending on which part of it you eat.

1. One needs to balance between eating just muscle meat and connective tissue. In other words, apart from eating steak, remember to include ligaments, tendons, silver skin in your diet. This is the gristle, which is usually discarded as it is difficult to cook and is tough and chewy when eaten if it is not cooked right.
2. Another area that needs balancing is in the ratio of protein to fat measured in calories. This is also known as Marcos which can get quite complicated. To keep it simple, animal fats such as tallow and lard can be used when cooking the meat to get the required ratio.
3. As mentioned earlier, eating different or all parts of the animal; muscle, organs, collagen, makes it possible to all the required vitamins and minerals.
4. Adding omega 3 fatty acids to your diet from liver, fish and seafood.

This combination should give your body all the nutrients it requires to function and keep you healthy and alive.

To measure the effects of the meat only diet on the body, keep track of your body weight, measurements, blood markers and body composition.

Background Of The Carnivore Diet

A Fad?

The large number of blogs and Youtube channels available on the internet make the Carnivore diet seem like a fad. The hosts seem like health fanatics trying to find any which way to get you on the diet, dropping medical statistics and benefits of eating just meat. They may be fanatical about it, but it is partially because they are seeing the results for themselves. They may also be fanatic because they are preaching to a crowd that is convinced that a balanced diet is the only way to get all the nutrients required by the body.

Even though there is currently no scientific data backing the carnivore diet, if we were to go back into history, we would find that there are cultures who ate almost nothing but meat. Not because they sat down and did a study about how many nutrients there are in meat compared to plants, but because they didn't have any other option as such. Take the Inuit of the Canadian Arctic whose staple diet is or was fish, seal, walrus and whale meat, or the Masaai of East Africa who were, and still are, sustained by meat, milk and blood. They ate what was available to them in their environment.

Historically

Georgia Ede MD on her website <u>Diagnosis Diet</u> shares a historical observation about vegan and carnivore diets to support this theory:

To the best of my knowledge, the world has yet to produce a civilization which has eaten a vegan diet from childhood through death, whereas there are numerous examples throughout recorded history of people from a variety of cultural, ethnic and geographical backgrounds who have lived on mainly-meat diets for decades, lifetimes, generations."

She shares a list of what she calls the "Meat Mongers" who are peoples whose diets were primarily carnivorous. The list includes
- The Inuit of the Canadian Arctic thrived on fish, seal, walrus and whale meat.
- The Chukotka of the Russian Arctic lived on caribou meat, marine animals and fish.
- The Masai, Samburu, and Rendille warriors of East Africa survived on diets consisting primarily of milk and meat.
- The steppe nomads of Mongolia ate mostly meat and dairy products.
- The Sioux of South Dakota enjoyed a diet of buffalo meat.
- The Brazilian Gauchos nourished themselves with beef.

The Maasai of East Africa

The Maasai are one of the few cultural groups who have maintained their traditional way of life in spite of the many advancements around them. They have maintained their traditional dress, their pastoralist and warrior lifestyle, and cultural rituals and ceremonies such as circumcision and rites of passage.

The Maasai, in Joram Arimi's <u>article</u>, to date predominantly consume what the modern world considers food high in cholesterol; meat milk and blood. The rural Maasai is a pastoralist and spends most of his time in the nomadic lifestyle searching for pasture for his cattle. He has no time to till the land because by the next season, it is time to move in search of new pastures of grass for the cattle. The Maasai live a very simple lifestyle with their main health issues are very basic, undernutrition, infectious diseases and child mortality. However, they do not suffer from any of the modern illnesses that dominate the lives of most urban dwellers.

As reported by Joram, although heart diseases are linked to high consumption of fat milk, the same milk is highly consumed by the rural Maasai. Interestingly, they do not have high levels of cholesterol as would be expected. This may be because they have to do a lot of walking on a daily basis; to find pasture for their cattle, to get firewood and fetch water. The amount of walking done by the Maasai on a given day would require one to spend a couple of hours in the gym to match. This walking probably contributes to burning off any excess calories that would be gained from their diet.

In addition to this, the Maasai include special herbs in the diet which have been proven to lower levels of cholesterol in the body. The bark of the magic gwarra, branches of the Jacket Plum, the root and bark of the East African green heart and thorn mimosa. When compared to his urban counterpart, the rural Maasai is much healthier as he does not indulge in the readily available processed carbohydrates; the white rice, white maize meal, white wheat flour, fried potatoes, cakes, bread and the like. When he does consume carbohydrates, he tends to boil them rather than fry them. The urban Maasai is less healthy and is showing signs of cholesterol and heart disease due to heavy indulgence in processed carbohydrates and reduced physical activity.

The Inuit of the Canadian Arctic

Due to the climatic conditions of the Arctic, it would be unwise to depend on agriculture as a source of food. The Inuit live a semi-nomadic lifestyle moving with the seasons where winter is spent on the sea, summers by the coast and spring further inland. To survive, they would hunt both on the land and in the sea, and like the Maasai, they too eat some of their meat raw and drink seal blood. They believed that eating meat was key to keeping them warm and making their bodies strong and healthy. What was happening in their body was that due to limited amounts of carbohydrates in the Inuit diet, the body would break down protein giving them consistent energy.

Where they lived and what they ate, depended on the season. During winter and summer, seals were the main source of food alongside fish and sometimes whale. Spring was the time to hunt the caribou and small birds. Other animals that they hunted included polar bear, walrus and the occasional whale which could feed a community for almost a year.

As the Inuit sometimes had to travel long distances to hunt for food, some of it would be eaten raw at the location of the kill. This was especially true for fish. With the seal, however, the whole community would share the seal. The hunters would get to eat first drinking some of the seal blood and eating choice parts of the liver, fat and the brain. Once the hunters had eaten, the rest of the community, the women and children, would get their share of what was left. This was not the regular eating habit of the Inuit as hunting did not result in a kill on a daily basis. On a regular day, they ate two main meals shared in a day and people eat when they are hungry. Most of their food is eaten either raw, frozen, fermented or boiled.

The modern world has come to the Inuit and much of their traditional way of life has changed. The no longer spend extended periods of time outdoors hunting or entertaining themselves with games. Technology has made the hunt easier as food is available at the convenience store and entertainment can be found on a screen.

Contradictions

These examples of traditional meat eaters have studies that support them and further studies that oppose them. Dr McDougall in his [2015 newsletter](#) states that misinformation about the Inuit diet was leading to dangerous eating habits. An advocate of the starch, vegetables and fruit diet on which he says humans thrive, the doctor is of the belief that the Inuit survived on just enough nutrition from their eating habits. That they were not the most healthy people but were making the best of a bad situation.

He goes on to justify that the Eskimo diet worked for them before the introduction of modern conveniences. Having to hunt for food and living in an igloo in extremely cold conditions helped to burn the calories that are gained from eating an all meat diet. Eating a similar diet today while living in a heated house, moving around in a car and getting all your shopping done at the supermarket leads to a sedentary lifestyle compared to that of the traditional Inuit. Coupled with the introduction of fast food, the all meat diet is a recipe for disaster.

But even without the modern conveniences, the Inuit suffer severe bone loss due to the low calcium diet and minimal sunshine, they were infected by the parasites that infected the wild animals they ate and, meat derived chemical pollution due to high levels of toxic, organic pollutants and heavy metal found in the meat of the sea animals they eat.

Such reports make it seem like there is no middle ground when it comes to diets and people's choice on what to eat or not eat. The Inuit ate what was available to them then, and doing the same today with the modern research about the balanced diet is not a good idea. The same with the Maasai, they lived in the way they knew best following what they believed worked for them.

Is The Carnivore Diet for Everyone?

As more and more people try out the carnivore diet, they are sharing their research and findings on YouTube and on their blogs. There are variations to the diet but the primary requirement remains meats with no carbohydrates, at least for the first days of the diet. After practising the strictly meat and water only dietary requirements for some time, people reintroduce some fruits and vegetables to their diet depending on how their body responds. Listening to different people, and their results it becomes clear that there are no fixed rules to this diet although there is the basic requirement that needs to be met to make it effective.

Many people argue that traditional meat eating people really didn't have a choice when picking their diet. They ate whatever was available and made the best of it, and that probably their bodies adapted to their environment and diet. They argue that this does not mean that everyone should adopt the same diet just because it seems to have worked for a particular community. Around the world, other communities have had access to a variety of foods including fruits and vegetables, some with more access to meat, others with less, and they still enjoyed excellent health.

Whichever way you look at it, the carnivore diet had challenged the notion that saturated fats and cholesterol cause heart disease. Both the Masaai and the Inuit show that through their diets were full of saturated fats and cholesterol, they were relatively free from heart disease and similar ailments until the introduction of modern processed foods. Both cultures were physically active; the Masaai looking for pasture for their animals, the Inuit going for long hunts, and they would spend extended periods of time outside.

Looking at the little evidence presented, going on the carnivore diet is a personal choice, as is how they choose to apply it. However so far, those who have tried it out report excellent health results and some have even made the choice to make the diet a lifestyle.

Today

Apart from the different cultures who had no choice as such but to eat a diet high in meat, there are those people whom due to counter the effects of an illness, found that the all meat diet worked wonders for them.

Mikhailah Peterson's blog starts with a statement that proposes that 'most health problems are treatable by diet alone'. Now in her mid-twenties, Mikhaila suffered juvenile rheumatoid arthritis from the age of seven which led to hip and ankle replacements. At age seventeen she was suffering depression, anxiety, insomnia and fatigue. After taking all types of drugs combined in different ways, in 2015 she stumbled on some research that showed that what she was eating was the primary cause of her discomfort. Profiled in the August 2018 UK publication The Times, she revealed how her diet of beef, salt and water relieved her of depression symptoms and all her other symptoms went into remission.

Dr Georgia Ede of Diagnosis:Diet found that changing her diet caused chronic fatigue, IBS and migraines to all but disappear. Now 52, she reports of a clean bill of health even though her family background is riddled with cases of obesity, diabetes, anxiety disorders and high cholesterol.

Amber O'Hearn has been on the carnivore diet for nine years and recommends it for people who have digestive problems, have an autoimmune disorder such as arthritis, asthma,skin problems such as eczema, mood disorders such as depression and the list goes on. She says she enjoys health at elevated levels from eat a carnivorous diet which she switched to after being on a low-carbohydrate diet for year. Within three weeks of being on the diet she lost weight she had gained from previous pregnancies and her depression had disappeared.

These are just a few of the many examples of the benefits people who have taken on the carnivore diet enjoy. While a majority of those taking up the diet are looking to lose weight and achieve a higher state of wellbeing, there really isn't any research on the positive or negative health effects of an all meat diet as such. Going forward there will be more data as those who have made the all meat diet a lifestyle record their results. But for now, we can only look to those who have tried it out and have found that the carnivore diet, when practised from the nose to tail, has reduced their symptoms of autoimmune conditions, made it possible to overcome chronic, severe health conditions such as Lyme disease, has uncovered food intolerances and has aided in weight loss.

Are There Really Health Benefits From Eating A Carnivore Diet?

Depending on who you are, and how you approach the diet, the benefits may vary. Ideally, when on the carnivore diet, one should not restrict themselves to eating just muscle meat. One should intentionally consume other parts of the animal such as bones, organs, skin which are very nutritious. When eating a well-balanced carnivore diet, there are some common benefits recorded:

1. The addiction to sweet things and cravings is pretty much eliminated.
2. Eating little or no carbohydrates causes your body to use stored fat for energy. This process is known as Ketosis and has been linked to benefits such as weight loss, strength gain, and reducing symptoms of mental illnesses such as ADHD.
3. Weight loss

Eating an imbalanced meat diet will eventually lead to a systematic amino acid imbalance which is linked to inflammation, lower lifespan and other problems. It can not be repeated enough, a true carnivore diet is not about eating just steak. Other parts of the animal must be included in the diet.

Sceptics abound and there are many people who have reported not seeing any benefits from going on the carnivore diet. When pressed, many of them did not stay on the diet long enough to see the results they have heard about. They got stuck at the transition stage and gave up. Others did not go full carnivore and cheated here and there. The largest group of sceptics are those whose minds are fixed on the traditional balanced diet and cannot imagine not eating carbohydrates and vegetables.

Considerations When Starting The Carnivore Diet

As you start the Carnivore diet, do not restrict yourself to certain amounts of meat or set times to eat. Eat when hungry and eat until full. Eating only proteins will change your usual eating habits considerably. Drink enough water but stay away from vegetable juices, energy drinks, soda, or protein shakes. Keep it as simple as possible. Also, reduce the amount of sugar in your tea or coffee should you choose to keep them in your diet. Resist the urge to add fruits or vegetables to your plate as this will defeat the purpose of the all meat diet.

Cook your meat to your taste and feel free to experiment. It may be difficult to take on meats that you are not used on eating on a regular basis and you may need a bit of direction and creativity.

When shopping for meat, it will be cheaper to buy in bulk. Your local butcher or farmer's market should be able to direct you. Do your best to avoid processed meats such as ham, salami and pepperoni. Take precautions when buying sausages as some suppliers use wheat to fill them out.

Good quality meat is definitely a plus. Where possible purchase meat from grass-fed or organically fed animals as this meat will be low in toxins from animal feeds laced with antibiotics, pesticides, GMO's, and other drugs.

Determine if you are taking up the diet short term or long term. How long you choose to do the Carnivore diet depends entirely on you. You could choose to take it up for a month to see how it works for you. If you like the results, you could consider making it a lifestyle.

Good quality meat tends to be expensive, therefore your budget is likely to increase significantly, however, food preparation becomes very simple. This is especially true for those with large families.

Transitioning

When you start the carnivore diet, your body initially rebels and suffers withdrawal symptoms from the foods it is accustomed to. This is the toughest period and the time when most people quit. This is where your will to improve your health so to speak is tested. If you can make it past this stage, you will enjoy the benefits of the carnivore diet.

The transition period could also be an indicator of how well, or how badly you have been eating. Those transitioning from Paleo or Ketogenic diets may barely feel the effects of the change in diet compared to those who are coming off the traditional 'balanced diet' which has large servings of carbohydrates. Those who snack a lot and binge on carbohydrates will have the hardest time transitioning.

Some of the indicators of this transition period include headaches, brain fog, nausea, diarrhoea, insomnia, muscle aches, low energy, irritability, and the list goes on. Changing one's diet comes at a price. The transition period varies from person to person. Some of the ways to shorten it include:
1. Eating more meat. When one is feeling under the weather, eating is the last thing on one's mind. However, the body needs fuel. Eat more.
2. Drink more water to keep hydrated.
3. Sleep. Allow your body to get some rest and heal itself.

4. Exercise. It seems contradictory to sleep, but exercising leads to sweating which helps rid the body of toxins.
5. Supplement on potassium, sodium, magnesium and chloride which your body is losing through all the sweating and peeing. Either drink bone broth or get a supplement.

The reason your body is reacting in this way is that is has become accustomed to burning sugar for energy. Now it has to adapt to burning fat for energy. This can be excruciating for those who have been on a high carbohydrate diet because the body behaves like it is recovering from an addiction.

Fewer carbohydrates in your diet mean your insulin levels drop. This is a sign to the kidneys that they need to release sodium which in turn means your body will also release a lot of water. All of this is part of the body adapting to burning fat for energy.

Effects On Your Body

1. Better Digestion

A balanced diet requires fibre which helps digestion. The carnivore diet proves the opposite. Your body handles digestion very well without the help of fibre. If anything, fibre upsets digestion causing bloating, gassiness and reduced bowel movement.

In 2010, the *World Journal of Gastroenterology* conducted a six-month study to investigate the effects of reducing the amount of fibre in people with chronic constipation. The participants of the study were required to avoid fibre for two weeks, after which they could slowly reintroduce it to their diets. Many of the participants reported excellent digestion and were reluctant to reintroduce fibre to their diet. Those who continued with fibre in their diet reported no change in their condition.

Steven R. Gundry, M.D has written a book titled *The Plant Paradox*, in which he states that have a natural defence mechanism that makes them unpalatable. The mechanism (lectins, gluten, phytic acid) causes digestive distress, bloating and gassiness which ought to lead to them being eaten less.

2. Mental Clarity

Those on the meat only diet report an increase in focus and mental clarity once the body had adjusted to getting energy from fats rather than carbohydrates. Without the dips and spikes caused by sugar, moodiness is reduced and one is better placed to handle stress. Studies carried out report that fewer carbohydrates and more protein and fats in one's diet have strong neuroprotective properties that help in improving focus.

3. Decreased Inflammation

A 2013 study recorded in the journal Metabolism compared people who ate a high-fat, low carbohydrate diet against people who ate a low-fat, high carbohydrate diet. Twelve weeks later, those on the high-fat diet recorded lower markers of systemic inflammation. The conclusion was that eating a high-fat diet may be good for overall cardiovascular health.

4. Faster Weight Loss

It would be expected that one would add weight from a meat only diet. However, due to the lack of carbohydrate, the body will maintain steady levels of blood sugar. When you eat carbohydrates the body tends to convert it to fat to counter blood sugar spikes caused by the carbohydrates. Removing carbohydrates from your diet will reduce the amount of fat created by your body.

Also, with minimal carbohydrates in your body, cravings will reduce and you will remain full for longer periods of time. Compulsive snacking will become a thing of the past.

5. Improved Testosterone

High-fat diets have been proven to increase testosterone levels. A study in the *American Journal of Clinical Nutrition* discovered that men on a high-fat, low-fibre diet for 10 weeks had a 13% higher testosterone compared to the men who were on a low-fat diet.

CHAPTER 2:
Starter Guide

The carnivore diet is pretty straight forward. Eat meat. However, it is important to know your meats. Take time to learn the different parts of the cow or pig so that you know which parts are most beneficial to providing your body with the nutrients it needs. For example, ribeye steak, back ribs, rib roast and porterhouse steak have more fat than sirloin and top round steak. This will guide your shopping and eating.

If you are able, purchase different cuts and types of meat for variety. Have a little white meat, some organs, red meat, fish and some eggs. This works for those who are gradually transitioning to the strict meat and water carnivore diet. Some people are comfortable remaining at this level of the diet as it works best for them.

It would be best to go cold turkey and suffer the transition period once and for all. However, you could also slowly condition your body by starting slow. Gradually cut out all carbohydrates, plant products and processed foods. As time goes on, and if you feel compelled to, you can go on to eat just meat.

Plan

You might want to take time off or spreading out your schedule the best you can for the first week of being on the carnivore diet. This is to accommodate the transition period. Rather than wait for it to hit you, prepare for it. Have a lot of water on hand, make time to sleep and exercise and allow your body to adapt with ease. Work-related or even personal stress is bound to make the transition period more difficult.

Have enough meat on hand as you will be hungry. Much as it would be great exercise, you really don't want to have to make a trip to the butcher when you are hungry. You might end up picking up a snack which is not part of the plan.

Set up a meal plan. This will take the stress out of having to think about what to prepare. It will also determine how you do your meat shopping. It simplifies things tremendously. You will eliminate standing in front of a fridge full of meat trying to figure out which meat to eat and how to cook it.

What Can You Eat?

To make life a little easier, here is a breakdown of what you can eat if you are not following the strict carnivore diet that requires you to eat only meat with salt, and drink water.

1. Red meat:

  Ground beef - Made into a patty and grilled or fried in tallow

  Steak cuts - Fried with sea salt

  Ground lamb

2. Organs:

  Liver

  Heart

  Tongue

3. White meat:

  Pork shoulder - pressure cooked

  Bacon

  Canned sardines packed in olive oil or water

  Wild salmon

  Canned mackerel

  Canned tuna

  Chicken wings wrapped in bacon made in the air fryer

  Chicken liver

4. Other:
> Free-range eggs
>
> Cheese, Goats cheese
>
> Butter (grass fed)
>
> Homemade tallow
>
> Homemade ghee from clarified butter
>
> Spices - can be reintroduced to the diet after 30 days of using only salt
>
> Sea salt
>
> Herbs - rosemary and thyme for lamb
>
> Onion and garlic
>
> Olive oil
>
> Black pepper

5. Drinks:
> Water,
>
> Sparkling water (with squeezed lemon)
>
> Coffee/Tea
>
> Herbal teas

Tips For Eating

It cannot be emphasised enough - eat when you are hungry. Do not wait for lunchtime or dinner time to eat. When the urge hits, dig in. If you are concerned about the nutritional value of the various types and cuts of meat, here are some well-known benefits of consuming various cuts of meat:

Benefits of Meat

Meat is high in protein. Many believe that a diet high in protein will affect your kidneys or leach calcium from your bones. As long as you are taking enough fluids, a high-protein diet will not affect your kidneys, and protein will not have a negative impact on bone health. Leaching is caused by phosphorus which is typically found in colas.

Red meat contains iron which is greatly required by adolescents, premenopausal and pregnant women.

Vitamin B12 found in animal products aids in digestion and energy production. Those who do not eat animal products are forced to take supplements to get this vitamin.

Keep in mind that the body handles saturated fats from processed meats and unprocessed meats differently. A few slices of deli meat full of nitrates and other preservatives will have an adverse effect on one's health compared to a steak from the local butcher.

Benefits of eggs

Eggs are often classified as dairy, however, they come from chicken and are high in protein, vitamin A, various B vitamins and minerals. Despite their high levels of cholesterol, they are safe and healthy to eat.

Benefits of Liver

Liver is a great source of essential amino acids, vitamins A, D, K, E, K12, iron and copper which are nutrients are necessary for a healthy body that can clean itself. These are many vitamins for one organ. To give an idea of how rich the liver is, here is a breakdown of the importance of a few of the vitamins and minerals found in it:

- Vitamin B12 helps the formation of red blood cells, healthy brain function and DNA
- Vitamin A helps the heart and kidney function and is important for vision, immunity and reproduction
- Iron helps to carry oxygen around the body
- Copper activates a number of enzymes which assist in the regulation of energy production, iron metabolism and brain function.

Benefits of Fish

Filled with omega-3 fatty acids, vitamin D and B2, fish is a low-fat high-quality protein. It is rich in calcium, phosphorus, iron, zinc, iodine, magnesium and potassium, nutrients that can lower blood pressure and reduce the risk of suffering from a heart attack or stroke. Omega-3 fatty acids are essential for heart and brain health and may decrease the risk of depression, dementia, diabetes, ADHD and Alzheimer's disease.

Pregnant women are advised to eat fish or take omega-3 supplements to facilitate healthy brain function and the development of infant vision and nerves.

Benefits of Bone Marrow

Considered a delicacy in many parts of the world, bone marrow is rich in nutrients. It is a good source of omega-3 fatty acids needed for healthy brain development and anti-inflammation

Benefits of Bone Broth

The bones used to make bone broth are rich in vitamins and nutrients such as calcium, magnesium, iron, vitamins A and K, fatty acids, zinc, manganese and phosphorus. Including connective tissue in the bone broth supplies the body with natural compounds and amino acids from the cartilage and the collagen.

When cooked, the collagen becomes gelatin which is important in helping protect joints from unnecessary stress. People with osteoarthritis may benefit from a reduction in pain, stiffness in the knee joints.

The amino acids aid in digestion, reducing inflammations in the body and promoting better sleep in some people.

High in protein, bone broth may support weight loss as it helps the body feel full for longer.

Benefits of Chicken

Chicken is a source of lean, low-fat protein and contains a variety of B vitamins, vitamin A and selenium. Rich in phosphorus, chicken is good for your teeth, bones, kidney, liver and central nervous system.

The benefits of these vitamins and nutrients are:

Vitamin B6 boots metabolism keeping energy high while burning away calories

Vitamin B2 takes care of skin problems

Selenium takes care of the thyroid, hormone, metabolism and immune functions

Serotonin amino acid which enhances moods

Vitamin A for healthy eyesight

Benefits of Lobster

100 grams of lobster meat will provide your body with Vitamin B12 taking care of your brain function, copper, omega-3, and other vitamins and minerals.

Benefits of Beef Heart

Beef heart is full of zinc, selenium, essential amino acids, phosphorus which are elements required by the body. Compared to other cuts of meat, beef heart has more than twice the amount of elastin and collagen.

CHAPTER 3:
Meal Plans & Recipes

Meal Plan

Depending on your appetite, you may have two, or five meals a day. Remember to eat when you are hungry, and eat until you are full.

Day One

Breakfast: Eggs, Bacon,

Lunch: Grilled Beef Liver

Dinner: Hamburger patties

Day Two

Breakfast: Bone Broth, leftover hamburger patties

Lunch: Chicken drumsticks

Dinner: Rib Eye

Day Three

Breakfast: Bacon Wrapped Salmon

Lunch: Grilled Lamb Chops

Dinner: Beef Heart Steak

Day Four

Breakfast: Eggs, Homemade Sausages

Lunch: Bone Broth, Grilled Shrimp

Dinner: Slow cooker Pork

Day Five

Breakfast: Leftover Pork, Bone Broth

Lunch: Pan- Fried Tilapia

Dinner: Herb Roasted Bone Marrow

RECIPES

Steak

Skillet Rib Eye

Ingredients
- 1 (1 1/4 pound) bone-in rib eye steaks (about 1 1/4 to 1 1/2-inch thick)
- 1 teaspoon of your favourite seasoning
- 2 teaspoons chopped fresh rosemary leaves
- 1 tablespoon unsalted butter
- 1 tablespoon olive oil

Instructions
1. Season the steak coating it evenly then sprinkle with the fresh rosemary leaves. Refrigerate for 2-3 days. When you are ready to cook your rib eye steaks, remove from the refrigerator in good time and allow to rest at room temperature for 30 minutes to remove the chill.
2. Heat a medium skillet over medium heat. Add a combination of the butter and olive oil to the skillet. As the butter melts, tilt the skillet from side to side to ensure that the whole pan is coated with the butter and olive oil.
3. Cook the ribeye on the skillet for five minutes or until the bottom of the steak is brown and caramelized. Turn it over and do the same. Using the butter and oil, and juices from the steak, baste the steak continuously until brown and caramelized or until it is cooked to your taste.
4. Remove the rib eye steak from the skillet allow to rest for a few minutes. Using a sharp knife, slice the steak against the grain. Remove the bone and serve.

Note:

To enhance the flavours of this steak, marinate it for 2-3 days. This will give it time to marinate well and be flavour-filled. Ensure that the seasoning you use is as natural as possible.

Olive Basted Strip Steak

Ingredients
- 3 tablespoons olive oil, divided
- 2 1 1/2-in.-thick strip steaks, trimmed
- 1 teaspoon kosher salt, divided
- 1 teaspoon freshly ground black pepper, divided
- 1 rosemary sprig
- 1 garlic clove, crushed

Instructions
1. Over medium-high heat the pan. While the pan is heating, season the steaks with salt and pepper, and brush with a tablespoon of oil.
2. Add a bit of the oil, the garlic and rosemary sprig to the pan. Add the steaks and cook for nine minutes or until cooked to one's taste, turning and basting regularly to ensure that both sides cook evenly.
3. Let the steaks rest for a few minutes on a cutting board before slicing against the grain. When serving, pour the juices from the skillet and cutting board on the steak and add more salt and pepper if necessary.

Note:

To keep the steaks moist, baste them after every turn. This also ensures that they cook evenly.

Brisket of Beef

Ingredients
- 16-pound first-cut beef brisket, trimmed so that a thin layer of fat remains
- 2 teaspoons all-purpose flour
- 1 pinch Freshly ground black pepper
- 3 tablespoons butter
- 8 medium onions, peeled and thickly sliced
- 3 tablespoons tomato paste
- 1 pinch Kosher salt
- 3 cloves garlic

Instructions
1. Heat the oven to 350°F and season the brisket with pepper.
2. In an ovenproof pot, heat the butter over medium-high heat. Add the brisket and brown until crusty in some areas, then put on a platter.
3. In the same pan, add the onions and stir continuously until the onions are soft and brown but not caramelised. Remove from the fire and put the brisket on top of the onions. Pour in any juices that have seeped from the brisket.
4. Spread the tomato paste over the brisket and season with salt and more pepper. Add the garlic and cover the pot. Bake in the oven for 1 ½ hours then remove from the pot and slice into ⅛ inch thick slices. Return the slices to the pot in the order they were sliced. Taste to check if it is well seasoned, and if necessary, add a bit of water to the pot, cover and return to the oven.
5. Reduce the heat to 325°F and cook for 1 ½ to 2 hours or until it is fork-tender. Check on it to ensure it is not drying up and to baste it. When cooked, serve with its juices.

Bacon Wrapped Steak

Ingredients
- 2 1 inch thick steaks
- 2 uncured bacon slices
- 2 Tbsp butter or ghee
- Sea salt and freshly ground black pepper
- Kitchen thread

Instruction
1. If your steaks were in the fridge, allow them to return to room temperature and pat them dry. Cut a length of thread long enough to circle the steak twice and tie a knot.
2. Wrap the bacon tightly around the steak shaping it into a roundish shape. Hold the bacon in place by tying the thread around the wrapped steak and fasten with a double knot.
3. Melt the butter or ghee in a small pan and gently add the bacon-wrapped steak. Cook each side on high heat for a few minutes depending on the thickness of the steaks and how you like them cooked. However, don't cook the steak to well-done or it will be dry and tough.
4. Serve immediately.

Bone Broth

Simple Bone Broth

Ingredients
- 1 gallon of water
- 1 ounce of vinegar
- 3–4 pounds of bones and tissues

Instructions
1. Put all the ingredients into a big pot or slow cooker then bring to the boil. Once it is boiling, reduce the heat to a simmer for 10-24 hours. After the broth is ready, you can strain out the bones and tissues, or leave them in and nibble at them as you drink the broth.

Notes:

You can add salt, pepper and natural spices for flavour. Consider adding in some vegetables for nutrients. Bones can be saved from other meals or bought from the butchery.

Ground Beef

Hamburger Patties

Ingredients
- 500g ground beef
- 1 egg, beaten
- 1 onion, diced (optional)
- Grated cheese
- Salt and pepper to taste
- 2 tablespoons butter

Instructions
1. Combine the ground beef, egg, onion, salt and pepper. Mix until the egg is completely incorporated. Separate the mixture into palm-sized balls and set aside.
2. Melt the butter on a pan. Place two or three meatballs, one at a time onto the pan and press down into a hamburger patty. Turn after a few minutes to ensure that they cook evenly. Serve immediately.

Notes:

The patties can be cooked on a grill, or left as meatballs and cooked in the oven.

Fish

The Best Garlic Cilantro Salmon

Ingredients
- 1 large salmon fillet
- 1 lemon
- 4 cloves of garlic, minced
- 1/4 cup fresh cilantro leaves, roughly chopped
- Kosher salt to taste
- Freshly cracked black pepper to taste
- 1 tbsp butter

Instructions
1. Turn on the oven to 400° F and line a baking sheet with foil. Put the fillet on the baking sheet, rub some butter on it, and squeeze lemon juice over it, and sprinkle the garlic, salt, pepper and cilantro on it.
2. Put the fillet in the oven and bake for about 10 minutes. Turn up the heat for a few minutes to bake the top to a crisp. Serve immediately.

Pan_Fried Tilapia

Ingredients
- 2 tilapia fillets
- salt to taste
- 2 tablespoons butter for frying

Instructions

Salt the tilapia fillets. Melt the butter on medium heat and place the fillets into the frying pan. Cook each side until the fish turns white. Turn only once so that the fish does not overcook and start to fall apart. Serve immediately

Sea Food

Grilled Split Lobster

Ingredients
- 2 tablespoons butter, plus more for the grill
- 2 1½-pound live lobsters
- Kosher salt and freshly ground black pepper
- Melted unsalted butter, hot sauce, and lemon wedges (for serving)

Instructions
1. Turn on the grill to medium-high heat.
2. Put the lobsters in the freezer for 15 minutes to slow down their nervous system and make it easier for you to cut them up.
3. With a kitchen towel, belly side down and head facing you, hold the tail and cut the lobster in half through the head and the body. Turn it around and cut through the tail. Remove any eggs or tomalley.
4. Rub the flesh side of the lobster with oil and season with salt and pepper. Press the fleshy side on the grill to cook for about 6-10 minutes. Turn and grill until the shells are slightly burned and the meat is cooked through.
5. Serve immediately with butter, hot sauce and lemon wedges.

Steam Your Own Lobster

Ingredients
- 4 lobster tails (approx. 1 lb with shell)
- Equipment – a steamer
- seasoning/ghee (optional)

Instructions
1. If the lobster tails are frozen, defrost them.
2. Set up the steamer, and bring the water to a boil. Place the lobster tails into the steamer and set your timer for 10 minutes. Fresh lobster can be steamed for a shorter time. Take the necessary precautions to keep from being scalded by the steam.

Grilled Shrimp

Ingredients

Shrimp Seasoning:
- 1 teaspoon garlic powder
- 1 teaspoon kosher salt
- 1 teaspoon Italian seasoning
- cayenne pepper to taste

For Grilling:
- 2 tablespoons extra virgin olive oil
- 1 tablespoon freshly squeezed lemon juice
- 1 pound shrimp — peeled and deveined
- Butter for the grill

Instructions

1. As the grill or oven is heating, mix together the seasoning ingredients. If you are using an oven, foil-wrap a baking sheet. Add the shrimp to the seasoning and ensure they are all coated. Grill or bake the shrimp until each side is cooked. Serve immediately.

Notes

Grilled shrimp is best eaten freshly cooked, although it can be refrigerated for up to 2 days.

Lamb

Grilled Lamb Chops

Ingredients
- 8 lamb chops 1 1/4 inches thick
- 3 tablespoons olive oil
- 2 tablespoons chopped fresh rosemary
- 3 cloves garlic minced
- 1 teaspoon kosher salt
- freshly ground black pepper to taste

Instructions
1. As the grill or oven is heating, combine the olive oil, rosemary, garlic, salt and pepper to make the marinade. Arrange the lamb chops next to each other on a plate and spread the marinade on both sides of the chops. Grill the chop for about 5 minutes each side, or until they are to one's taste. Transfer to a platter when cooked and allow to rest for 10 minutes before serving.

Liver

Skewer Grilled Liver Kebabs

Ingredients
- 1.1 lbs liver
- 1 tsp cayenne pepper optional
- 1 tsp ground cumin
- 1 tsp salt
- skewers

Marinade
- 1 tsp salt
- 1 tbsp ground sweet paprika
- 1/2 tsp ground cumin

Instructions
1. The day before, cut the liver into cubes ¾ inch thick. Combine the salt, sweet paprika and cumin to make the marinade. Mix in the liver, and leave overnight in the fridge.
2. Light up the grill as you put the liver cubes on the skewers. Don't put too many cubes on the skewers.
3. Grill the liver, turning frequently to ensure that they cook evenly. Once the liver is cooked through, serve immediately sprinkled with the cumin, salt and cayenne powder.

Grilled Beef Liver

Ingredients
- 1 lb beef liver cut into thin slices
- ½ cup olive oil
- 1 garlic clove crushed
- 1 tbsp fresh mint finely chopped
- 1 tsp salt
- ¼ tsp black pepper freshly ground

Instructions
1. Wash the liver and cut out any tough veins, and cut into thin slices. Mix together the olive oil, mint, salt, pepper and garlic in a bowl. Put in the liver slices and cover well.
2. As the liver is marinating, preheat a large grill pan over medium-high heat.
3. Grill the slices for about 10 minutes turning the slices to ensure they are cooked on both sides. Serve immediately.

Bacon-wrapped Liver With Sage

Ingredients
- 1 package of good-quality bacon
- 1 pound of chicken livers
- 3 tablespoons fresh sage

Instructions
1. While the oven is heating to 450°F, clean and cut the liver into small pieces. Cut the bacon strips to the length required to cover a piece of liver. Wrap the liver together with a piece of sage with a bacon strip and pierce with a skewer or toothpick to hold in place.
2. Bake until bacon is brown and crispy, and the liver is cooked, or for about 25 minutes. Serve warm.

Pan-Fried Liver

Ingredients
- 500g liver
- Butter
- Salt
- Pepper

Instructions

Clean the liver, and cut into palm-sized pieces. Melt the butter in a pan on medium-high heat. Add as many pieces of the liver that can fit, and let them cook slowly. Turn the pieces over to ensure that they cook evenly. When the liver is cooked, season with salt and pepper and serve warm.

Heart

Beef Heart Steak

Ingredients
- 1 tablespoon ghee
- 4 slices of beef heart 1" thick
- ¼ cup apple cider vinegar or plain milk
- 2 tablespoon rosemary infused olive oil (or plain olive oil)
- salt and pepper to taste

Instructions
1. Marinate the beef heart in either ¼ cup apple cider vinegar or plain milk for 24 hours. Put some ghee on a skillet and put on high heat. As you put the slices of heart on the skillet, they should sizzle. Cook on each side until browned on the outside but still pink on the inside. Sprinkle the olive oil over the cooked meat and serve warm.

Bacon

Bacon Wrapped Salmon

Ingredients
- 2 fillets of salmon
- 4 slices of bacon
- 1 Tablespoon of olive oil
- 2 Tablespoons of tarragon to garnish
- Lemon wedges, to serve

Instructions
1. Set the oven to 350°F (180°C) and wrap the salmon fillets with the bacon. Arrange on a roasting tray and sprinkle with olive oil, and bake for around 20 minutes. Serve warm, topped with chopped tarragon and lemon wedges.

Bacon and Beef Heart Rolls

Ingredients
- 12 oz Beef Heart meat, trimmed and sliced into 1" thick pieces
- 12 Bacon Slices
- ¼ teaspoon garlic powder
- ¼ teaspoon dried parsley
- ¼ teaspoon dried chilli flakes
- ½ teaspoon Sea Salt
- Toothpicks soaked in water

Instructions
1. Turn on the oven. In a bowl, combine garlic powder, dried parsley, chilli flakes and salt. Roll the pieces of heart in the mixed seasoning and cover evenly.
2. Use the bacon strips to wrap the beef heart pieces and hold in place with the soaked toothpicks. Place the beef and bacon rolls in the oven and bake until the bacon turns brown and is crispy, or a little longer depending on how well done you want the beef heart to be.
3. Serve immediately

Chicken

Crispy Indian Drumsticks

Ingredients
- 10 chicken drumsticks
- 2-3 Tablespoons salt
- 3-4 Tablespoons garam masala or other spice
- 1/2 Tablespoon of coconut oil

Instructions
1. Turn on the over to 450F (230C) and use the oil to grease a baking tray. In a bowl, mix together the salt and garam masala. Evenly coat each drumstick with the seasoning and place on the baking tray spaced well. Bake for about 45 minutes or until the skin is brown and crispy, and the meat is pulling away from the bottom of the drumstick.

Roast Chicken

Ingredients
- 1 whole chicken
- 2 sprigs rosemary
- 2 garlic cloves
- 1 tablespoon coarse sea salt
- 1 teaspoon mixed herbs

Instructions
1. If the chicken has been in the fridge, give it time to come to room temperature and clean it. Preheat oven to 350 F and place the chicken, breast up, on a baking tray.
2. Fill the cavity with the rosemary and garlic, then sprinkle the mixed herbs and salt evenly over the whole chicken.
3. Bake for about an hour and a half depending on the size of the chicken and how hot your oven is.
4. To confirm that the chicken is cooked, the leg should separate from the body with ease, the meat should not be pink, and any juice should be clear. Serve warm.

Pork

Slow Cooker Pork

Ingredients
- 2 lb pork shoulder
- Salt to taste
- 1 tablespoon ginger powder
- 1 tablespoon peppercorns (or choice seasoning)

Instructions
1. Place the pork, uncut, into the slow cooker and pour the mixed seasoning evenly over the meat.
2. Set slow cooker for 8 hours on the low heat setting. After about 4-5 hours, carefully turn over the meat without pulling it apart.

Bone Marrow

Herb Bone Marrow

Ingredients
- Marrow bones
- Fresh rosemary
- Fresh thyme
- Salt and black pepper

Instructions
1. Thaw the bones if frozen. Set the oven to 400F. Chop the rosemary and thyme and mix together with salt and pepper. Arrange the bones on a baking tray and sprinkle with the freshly chopped herb combination. Bake for about 20 minutes or until the insides are not pink. Serve hot.
2. Leftover marrow can be used to add flavour to sauces and other meals.

Links

Everyday Health https://www.everydayhealth.com/diet-nutrition/diet/carnivore-diet-benefits-risks-food-list-more/

Biohackers https://www.biohackerslab.com/all-meat-diet-plan/

Healthy Home Economist https://www.thehealthyhomeeconomist.com/carnivore-diet/

http://www.learnalberta.ca/content/ssognc/inuitLifestyle/index.html

https://en.wikipedia.org/wiki/Inuit_cuisine

Mike Fishbein https://mfishbein.com/carnivore-diet/

https://meat.health/knowledge-base/carnivore-diet-symptoms-and-cures/

https://perfectketo.com/carnivore-diet/

https://www.acefitness.org/education-and-resources/lifestyle/blog/6602/the-health-benefits-of-the-right-kinds-of-meat

https://www.onnit.com/academy/the-carnivore-diet/

https://www.healthline.com/nutrition/why-liver-is-a-superfood#section7

https://www.doh.wa.gov/CommunityandEnvironment/Food/Fish/HealthBenefits

https://www.medicalnewstoday.com/articles/323903.php

http://www.peacockspoultryfarm.com/cooking/the-health-benefits-of-eating-chicken/

https://en.wikipedia.org/wiki/Plant_defense_against_herbivory

https://www.sciencedaily.com/terms/plant_defense_against_herbivory.htm

https://www.kevinstock.io/health/health-dangers-of-eating-seeds/

http://www.empiri.ca/p/eat-meat-not-too-little-mostly-fat.html

Manufactured by Amazon.ca
Bolton, ON